Contents

Acknowledgements

I am most grateful to the the authors and researchers of the all the works I have referred to for their efforts in helping us to understand the nature of the world and for highlighting the areas where our knowledge is incomplete.

I gratefully acknowledge Dr. Peter Briggs, of the British Association for the Advancement of Sciences, for permission to print the graph *England and Wales: Deaths of Children under 15 years attributed to scarlet fever, diphtheria, whooping cough and measles* (© Porter 1971).

I should like to thank Liz Benedict for asking for the information; Topper Browne for helping me to find it; Francesca Swainston for the initial encouragement to put pen to paper; Sharon Dorell for editing my flights of fancy and Ian Watson for making the final book possible.

Trevor Gunn
Brighton, 1992

Introduction

Immunisation has been practised for over a century and we have been led to believe that it has been responsible for the decline of infectious disease, and is effective in disease prevention.

However, a small but growing section of the community have vigorously opposed the use of vaccines. Many people have refused immunisations for themselves and their children, some doctors have refused to administer vaccines, and several pharmaceutical companies have ceased their manufacture.

To obtain an accurate assessment of the effectiveness of any medical treatment, relevant comparisons of results have to be made. Results from treated and untreated individuals, using as large a sample group as possible, covering a sufficiently long period of time, and taking into account as many of the influencing factors as possible.

The information presented here has been collated from the results of such investigations. They appear to indicate that the claims for the effectiveness of immunisation are not only unfounded but also mislead the general public into accepting a treatment that may be very damaging to our health.

The Germ Theory of Disease

The orthodox view maintains that infectious diseases are caused by specific micro-organisms. These are conditions which, in the past, left doctors with little or no effective means of treatment other than symptomatic relief, for example replacing fluids in conditions of severe vomiting and diarrhoea, body cooling for extreme fever, and pain relief.

The logical step towards an effective treatment would seem to be to try and combat the action of these micro-organisms in the body and to avoid infection by contamination. Through the development of antibiotics and vaccines this appears to have been partly achieved.

The Immune Response

Under normal circumstances in the body, foreign particles, such as bacteria and viruses, are recognised by specialised cells known as the *immune cells*. The immune cells function by producing *antibodies* that are able to attach to foreign particles present, rendering them harmless.

The antibodies fit on to specific sites on each particle just as a key would fit a lock. The initial response to infection would seem to be the production of the correct key to fit the specific lock, i.e. the correct antibody for the particular foreign particle present.

During this phase, one would usually experience the symptoms of that particular infectious disease. For example, fever, malaise and the appearance of red blotches are the usual symptoms of measles and these occur when measles virus is active in the body. It would appear that once sufficient antibodies have been produced, the measles virus is inactivated and the patient recovers.

These antibodies remain in the body and are able to recognise subsequent infections of the same (or similar) micro-organisms and are more able to cope with their elimination without producing all the symptoms of the disease.

Thus, a person who has suffered from an infectious disease is less likely to succumb to a second bout of infection, and is said to be *immune*. This type of protection is known as *acquired immunity*.

What is a Vaccine?

A vaccine is a special preparation of bacterial or viral particles which are similar to those thought to be responsible for the disease. However, these particles must be *attenuated*, in other words, prepared in some way which reduces their harmful properties.

The vaccine is said to mimic the disease and, when injected into the blood stream, the immune cells of the body are stimulated into producing antibodies against the specific vaccine components. These antibodies remain in the body and are able to recognise these or similar micro-organisms should any future infections occur.

Because of the method of vaccine preparation, the vaccine particles should not have any harmful effects and do not therefore produce the associated symptoms of disease.

For example, a measles vaccine may contain inactivated (i.e. killed) measles virus, which would stimulate the immune cells into producing antibodies to the measles virus when injected into the blood stream. There are no symptoms of measles because the virus has been previously inactivated, yet the antibodies remain in the body and theoretically protect the person from further infection.

We thus appear to have antibody production and immunity from a vaccine, without having to suffer the symptoms of the disease. This is known as *artificial immunity*.

Immunisation is said to be:

The only effective means of preventing (potentially) dangerous infectious diseases and epidemics.

Primarily responsible for the decline in infectious diseases.

Relatively harmless compared to the risk of serious disorders arising from infectious diseases.

However, the difficulty in vaccine preparation is in the production of vaccine micro-organisms that are sufficiently similar to the active micro-organisms thought to be responsible for the disease.

If inactivation of the vaccine micro-organisms changes them markedly from their original active state, then the antibodies produced do not respond to active micro-organisms in the real disease situation ..... the key does not fit the lock.

On the other hand, if the vaccine micro-organisms are not sufficiently altered (in the inactivation process), they may produce the very symptoms and complications one is trying to avoid in the real disease situation, or they may in fact be more dangerous.

The Germ Theory in Question

There is a growing body of evidence which suggests that disease is not caused primarily by external agents. Bacteria and viruses, in disease situations, are in fact the *end result* of a disease process which started some time earlier.

In the 19th century Antoine Bechamp recognised the influence of live particles in disease processes. At the same time Louis Pasteur, now famous for pioneering research into germ theory, explained these processes in terms of 'spontaneous generation.'[1] That means, he believed that life and the associated processes of decomposition and sepsis spontaneously emerge from nothing, a popular doctrine in the 19th century .

On seeing the results of Bechamp's work, Pasteur formulated his germ theory of disease, whereby disease is thought to be caused by the introduction of micro-organisms into the body from an external source.

However, Bechamp went on to show that these particles (bacteria and viruses, among others) were *already present* within normal cells, and that there need be no infection from outside of the body to cause disease. Any collection of cells could initiate fermentation, decay and disease by virtue of the particles already present in the cell structure.

Thus, the theories explaining the cause of disease split into the so-called orthodox and alternative views. The orthodox view maintains that disease starts with the introduction of micro-organisms into the body. The alternative theory is that the body degenerates into a diseased state *first,* and subsequently allows the proliferation of bacteria and viruses.

Micro-Organisms: The *Results* of Disease

Genetic Influences

The function of a cell is largely controlled by the *cellular genes*. These are the information centres of a cell, controlling the production of the cell building-blocks and the components involved in cell *metabolism*. The process of metabolism is concerned with the biochemical reactions which influence what the cell produces, how it functions, what fuels it uses and its chemical and electrical activity.

A cell contains many genes, only some of which are 'switched on' at any one time. The function of a particular gene is pre-programmed and may not change, and these are our inherited characteristics.

However, certain factors do influence the switching on or off of genes, factors such as hormones, nutrients and toxins. Normally genes function in maintaining the health of a cell and hence the entire body, but under certain conditions some cellular genes can be activated to bring on the symptoms of disease. For example, certain toxins can switch on genes that cause cancer, genes that were previously dormant but nevertheless present in normal cells.

Experiments have shown that by altering the chemical medium of cells it is possible to produce all the symptoms of a disease without introducing viruses or bacteria.

Bechamp first recognised the activity of certain cellular particles in disease processes, and these were later shown to be *chromatin particles,* which contain the cellular genes.

His observations show how disease and associated symptoms can be brought about by the activity of genes that are normally present within cells, this activity being under the influence of hormones, nutrients and toxins.

Bacteria

Bacteria are small, single-celled organisms, many of which inhabit the body. They perform a range of activities necessary for our healthy functioning. Like genes, bacteria are under the influence of their surrounding environment, and their activity will vary according to the hormonal, nutritional and toxic state of the body in which they are found.

Experiments have shown that it is possible to change bacteria from one type to another by altering their nutritional surroundings, i.e. from bacteria that normally maintain health to those that have pathological effects (producing symptoms of disease).[2]

For example, the same intestinal bacteria necessary for digestion in humans can, under certain conditions of poor nutrition, be changed into the destructive bacteria of typhoid, (bacillus coli to bacillus typhus), an apparently reversible process.[3]

Viruses

Viruses are generally much smaller than bacteria and are basically single units composed of genetic material in a protective coating. In order to reproduce themselves viruses need to take over the functions of the cell in which they are found, known as the *host cell*. This they do by interacting with the cellular genes, therefore active viruses are generally detrimental to the host cell.

Findings published in 1955 emphasised the structural similarities between viruses and genes.[4] Some viruses may be described as aberrant gene particles produced from the destruction of cells.

The observation of cell viruses in diseased tissue may be suggestive of previous cell damage, rather than indicating disease caused by infecting viruses.

Similarly, as with bacteria, viruses can change from one form to another by altering the media upon which they grow. A previously harmless viral particle can change into a pathological virus, (one producing symptoms of disease), simply due to the nutritional changes of its surroundings.[5]

Summary

It has been shown that disease conditions can arise from normal tissue components (genes, bacteria or viruses) due to changes within cells, and that there need be no infection by external micro-organisms to cause disease.

What are the Real Causes of Disease?

Traditionally it was thought that micro-organisms cause disease, yet most individuals have bacteria and viruses present within them that do no harm. In many cases these same particles are necessary for maintaining healthy cells.

However, when the cellular environment changes (due to toxins, poor nutrition or chemical changes from mental and emotional stress), these particles become *pathogenic* (disease-producing). At this stage, external micro-organisms are able to infect and proliferate, thus causing secondary complications. These infecting micro-organisms are not, however, the cause of the original condition.

Antimicrobial treatment (designed to kill microbes such as bacteria) may help in the final stages of disease, where patients are mainly suffering the effects of the pathogenic micro-organisms. However, with such treatment, there is a danger of neglecting the real causes of the disease, and whilst some symptoms may be alleviated for a period of time, often the complaint will recur. This is because the end result is being treated and not the pre-condition.

Antimicrobial treatment also has the effect of destroying the natural balance of micro-organisms within the body, as not only will the so-called harmful bacteria be destroyed, but many of the necessary health-conferring organisms will be eliminated also. This allows harmful organisms to grow and flourish where they otherwise would not.

This effect is not only confined to the original site of 'infection', but can also occur elsewhere in the body at the same time. Candidiasis (thrush), for example, is a fungal infection of the mouth, respiratory tract and vagina which commonly occurs after any kind of antibiotic treatment.

Such treatment may also leave the individual more susceptible to other diseases, some of which may be more serious than the original complaint. For example, the antibiotic treatment of childhood throat infections can lead to prolonged and frequent bouts of the original complaint. In addition, as a result of the treatment, the child may now be susceptible to more serious chest infections which require further doses of antibiotics. Similarly, the antibiotic treatment of bladder infections may lead to recurrence of the original problem plus a greater susceptibility to more serious kidney infections.

The real causes of disease are a combination of factors such as inherited tendencies, pollution, sanitation, diet, drug habits and mental or emotional stress, all of which affect people according to their own particular susceptibility.

Many therapies, by stimulating the natural self-healing capacity of the body or by addressing the nutritional and toxic condition of the body are able to reverse disease conditions. The cellular environment is no longer supportive to the pathogenic micro-organisms, the person is restored to health, and there has been no need to use toxic materials to kill micro-organisms.

Epidemics do not support the Germ Theory

Infectious diseases have replaced each other in time according to the level of health of the population. For example in England, before the introduction of vaccinations and antibiotics, plague gave way to typhus, typhus to smallpox, and smallpox to measles. In all cases the severe disease gave way to a less severe one as general living conditions improved.

Deaths from tuberculosis, smallpox, typhus, and typhoid had already declined by 90%, from approximately 6000 per million of population in 1860 to under 1000 per million in 1940, *before* the introduction of antibiotics and compulsory immunisation in England and Wales.[6]

Furthermore, epidemics are restricted by the conditions that support them. People who live in neighbouring areas or who pass through epidemic areas very rarely contract the disease, even though they are exposed to the micro-organisms associated with that disease.

However, if a susceptible individual is exposed to these conditions for long enough, the likelihood of contracting the disease will increase. It is also worth bearing in mind that, in so-called epidemic conditions, the vast majority of the people in that area do not succumb to the disease. This is illustrated by the fact that in the U.S.A. only 35 cases per 100,000 population warrants classification as a polio epidemic.[7]

Are there benefits in aseptic surgery?

If micro-organisms do not cause disease, why has aseptic (free from micro-organisms) surgery brought about such dramatic reductions in the incidence of wound infection?

When unclean or putrefying matter enters an open wound, morbid micro-organisms (those associated with disease) are introduced, along with a decaying substance. This alters the normal functions of the inherent micro-organisms and of cell metabolism, thus providing a soil on which these micro-organisms can grow and proliferate.

General cleanliness that automatically follows aseptic technique has been the major factor in reducing wound infection. Specific antibacterial air sprays have been found ineffective.[8] Micro-organisms cannot cause infection unless they find their own particular morbid soil in which to feed and grow. Airborne micro-organisms very often fail to produce infectious conditions, even in open wounds.

These conclusions have been further reinforced by a drugs watchdog committee report of 1991.[9] This report stated that salty fluids or even tap water may be better for clean wounds than commercial antiseptic preparations, as in some cases antiseptics can slow down the healing process. The Drugs and Therapeutics Bulletin sent to doctors recommends that some products should be banned by the Medicines Control Agency because they do more harm than good.

The report goes on to say how certain antiseptics may have a useful role where wounds are dirty or infected, but there is no evidence that antibiotic ointments or powders are of any value in these situations..... *'The widespread use of such products on wounds and ulcers is scientifically unjustified...'*

This further illustrates the importance of cleanliness and the 'soil' of infection, rather than the presence of micro-organisms and the need to destroy them. It also provides us with an example of how an ineffective treatment can become widely accepted and extensively used based solely on a supposedly scientific theory (germ theory). The antibiotic treatment of wounds has often been quoted as being scientifically justifiable but in reality it has not gone through the rigours of scientific analysis in real life situations.

Why was the Germ Theory so Popular?

Walene James gives the following factors as some of the main reasons for the popularity of the germ theory:[10]

Ideas on germ theory seem to fit human nature - man has apparently been ever ready to avoid responsibility for himself and was far more willing to place the blame on the bad micro-organisms that flew about and attacked him.

The theory was also congruent with the mechanistic theories of the universe more popular in the 19th century.

And, perhaps the most important reason - its great commercial value.

If we accept that micro-organisms can cause disease, treatments can be developed which counteract them. If disease is a result of a combination of diet, sanitation, and mental health fewer people would be able to make financial gain. Cure would appear to lie in the hands of the individual and the authorities concerned with environmental standards.

In spite of all the evidence supporting the alternative view of health and disease, is it possible to obtain some beneficial effect from immunisation?

Current Evidence - Does Immunisation Work?

Prior to the introduction of vaccinations there were no clinical trials carried out to measure the efficacy of vaccines in preventing disease - their clinical justification was, and still is, purely their ability to produce an antibody response.

Assuming that certain vaccines succeed in stimulating the body into producing certain antibodies, this still leaves many questions unanswered:

Are immunised people any less likely to contract the disease as unimmunised people, in other words, does an antibody response equal immunity?

How long does immunity conferred by vaccination last?

Are immunised people healthier than unimmunised individuals or are they more likely to contract other, more serious diseases?

What are the adverse effects of immunisations in both the short term and the long term?

Is natural immunity safer, longer lasting, and more effective?

One way to approach these questions is by analysing populations of immunised and unimmunised individuals. In doing so, one must ask whether any other factors are involved, and what are the controls (the control group being an unimmunised group from which comparisons can be made).

Poliomyelitis

The case of polio is of particular interest since its apparent decline cannot be explained by improvements in sanitation or diet. It is a disease that occurs only in the apparently more developed countries. There have been three polio epidemics in the U.S.A. this century. The first two simply declined at a time when there was no available treatment. In the late 1940's the decline of the third epidemic was credited to the polio vaccine (Salk vaccine).

The North Carolina Health Department's claims for the efficacy of the Salk vaccine showed that from 1953 to 1957, polio had decreased from 15,600 cases to 2,499 cases. However, during the 1962 congressional hearings, Dr. Bernard Greenberg, Head of the Department of Biostatistics of the University of North Carolina School of Public Health, testified that not only did the incidence of polio *increase* substantially (50% and 80% respectively during the years 1957-8 and 1958-9) after the introduction of mass immunisation programmes, but that the statistics had been manipulated to give the opposite impression.

The evidence given was as follows:

It was not until 1955 that a single person was given a polio vaccine injection. A 61% decrease in polio cases in 1954 was credited to the Salk vaccine when it was not even available in the state!

There was a redefinition of the term epidemic. More cases were required to qualify as an epidemic after the introduction of the Salk vaccine (from 20 per 100,000 head of population to 35 per 100,000).

There was redefinition of the disease. In order to be classified as suffering from paralytic poliomyelitis the patient had to exhibit symptoms for at least 60 days. Prior to1954, patients had to exhibit symptoms for only 24 hours.

There was mislabelling of diseases. After the introduction of the Salk vaccine, cocksackie virus and aseptic meningitis had been distinguished from paralytic poliomyelitis, in other words polio cases were now being called by a different name. In addition, non-paralytic polio cases were now reported as viral or aseptic meningitis.

Since the period 1955 to 1966 the incidence of polio has declined steadily, but viral and aseptic meningitis has increased. In 1975 it was reported that polio showed a count of zero, while a footnote explained that all such cases were now reported as meningitis.[11]

Not only does the Salk vaccine appear to have had no effect in the prevention of polio, but the evidence points to mass inoculation against polio being the *cause* of most of the remaining cases of the disease and in September 1977, John Salk, who developed the killed polio virus vaccine, testified along with other scientists to that effect. He said that most of the polio cases since the 1970's probably were a product of the live polio vaccine in standard use.[12]

Smallpox

The decline in incidence of smallpox has long been heralded as a triumph of vaccination. However, a closer look at the results reveals otherwise.

In England, free vaccinations were introduced in 1840 and made compulsory in 1853, yet between 1857 and 1859 there were 14,244 deaths from smallpox. After a population rise of 7%, the death rate rose by 40.8% to 20,059, between 1863 and 1865. In 1867 evaders of vaccination were prosecuted. Those left unvaccinated were very few. After a population rise of 9%, the death rate from smallpox rose by 123% to 44,840, between 1870 and 1872.[13]

In the Philippines, the largest smallpox epidemic occurred between 1917 and 1919, in which there were 162,503 cases and 71,453 deaths. All cases were vaccinated.[14]

In Japan, after the introduction of compulsory vaccination in 1872, the incidence of smallpox increased every year. In 1892 there were 165,774 cases and 29,979 deaths, all of whom were vaccinated.[15]

In the United Kingdom, the Department of Health admitted that whether or not a person has been vaccinated determines the diagnosis of subsequent diseases. This means that a person vaccinated against smallpox is 'protected' and if they subsequently contract the disease it will be diagnosed as something else (examples include chickenpox, pustular eczema, varioloid and monkeypox).[16]

In the 30 years up to 1934, 3,112 people are stated to have died of chickenpox and only 579 of smallpox in England and Wales, yet all authorities are agreed that chickenpox is a non-fatal disease.[17]

Professor Zuckerman, of the World Health Organisation Advisory Panel on Viruses, warned against the smallpox vaccine, indicating the prevalence of monkeypox which, according to the weekly epidemiological record of the W.H.O., is clinically indistinguishable from smallpox. As with poliomyelitis, smallpox cases are now being called by a different name.

Whooping cough

There is a tendency to under report the incidence of whooping cough in vaccinated children and to over report the incidence of the disease in unvaccinated children.[18] For example, in the U.S.A. the television programme, *D.P.T. - Vaccine Roulette*, shown in April 1982, warned of the dangers of vaccination. Within months, whooping cough epidemics were reported in the states of Maryland and Wisconsin.

It was stated by the Maryland Health Officials that the 'epidemic' was due to parents seeing the documentary and not having their children vaccinated. The cases were analysed by J. Anthony Morris, an expert on bacterial and viral diseases. In Maryland, 5 of the 41 cases were confirmed; all of them had been vaccinated. In Wisconsin, 16 of the 43 cases were confirmed; all of them had been vaccinated.[19]

In Sweden, the decline in incidence and deaths from whooping cough continued on its pre-vaccination level of decline even after the introduction of the whooping cough vaccine, i.e. the vaccine did not appear to cause any further decrease in incidence. It was later decided to withdraw the vaccine because of the mounting evidence implicating it as the cause of effects ranging from slight neurological damage to paralysis and death. The decline in incidence and the number of deaths from whooping cough continued to fall at exactly the same rate even though the vaccine was no longer widely available.[20]

Dr. Gordon Stewart, Head of the Department of Community Medicine, University of Glasgow, is a vigorous critic of the pertussis (whooping cough) vaccine. He has witnessed many outbreaks of the disease in vaccinated children and said ......'now in Glasgow 30% of our whooping cough cases are occurring in vaccinated patients' and 'the decline in pertussis mortality was 80% before the vaccine was ever used'. He also shares the view that the key factor in controlling whooping cough is probably the improvement in living conditions of potential victims.

Diphtheria

Cook County Hospital in Illinois immunised one half of its nursing staff against diphtheria. Soon after, diphtheria broke out in the immunised staff and not the others. It later affected both the immunised and unimmunised alike, the total number of cases being much higher amongst the immunised group.[21]

Following the introduction of compulsory immunisation, the incidence of diphtheria *increased* by 30% in France, 55% in Hungary, it tripled in Switzerland and increased from 40,000 per year to 250,000 in Germany, mostly affecting immunised patients. On the other hand, in Sweden diphtheria virtually disappeared without any recourse to immunisation.[22]

Rubella (German Measles)

This illness in children does not usually require medical treatment other than rest and adequate fluid intake. If contracted during the first three months of pregnancy, however, it can lead to damage of the unborn child. Immunisation is therefore only useful if the conferred immunity lasts from the time of immunisation up to childbearing age.

A study by the University of Minnesota showed that a large proportion of children had no evidence of immunity four to five years after vaccination.[23] In another study, 80% of army recruits immunised against rubella subsequently contracted the disease.[24]

Prior to the introduction of vaccines an estimated 85% of adults were naturally immune to rubella.[25] Today, the vast majority of women never acquire natural immunity. If their vaccine-induced immunity wears off they may be more likely to contract rubella whilst pregnant.

The concern of a group of doctors, led by two eminent epidemiologists in Connecticut, succeeded in having rubella struck from the list of legally required immunisations in the state.[26]

Measles

Measles is essentially a mild childhood disease with very few or no complications in the vast majority of cases. However, some individuals do develop serious problems such as encephalitis (inflammation of the brain), which can be fatal. The risk of encephalitis is a major factor which is cited to justify the use of measles vaccine.

Recent evidence suggests that between one in a thousand and one in five thousand children who contract measles naturally may develop encephalitis, and in later years between one in five thousand and one in a million may develop subacute sclerosing pamencephalitis (SSPE)[27]. However, other factors do play an important role in the development of encephalitis and measles-associated deaths, such as serious head injuries, close exposure to certain animals, poor nutrition and failure to treat complications[28].

The real risks of serious complications arising from contracting measles in the average child may be extremely small, and without the necessary contributory factors most children may not be at risk at all. Furthermore, the measles vaccine itself can cause encephalitis and subsequent death - the particular strain of measles virus used in the vaccine has been isolated from the spines of victims, proving that the vaccine caused the encephalitis[29].

A study in West Germany reported that one in 17,650 individuals vaccinated against measles developed temporary encephalitis and one in 2,500 had neurological complications[30]. Furthermore, doctors admit that notified side-effects of the vaccine are an under-estimate of the true number.

How Effective is the Measles Vaccine: Do the Benefits Outweigh the Risks?

In the U.S.A. the measles vaccine has been available since 1957 and the triple vaccine against measles, mumps and rubella (MMR) has been available since 1975. In spite of this, from 1983 to 1990 there has been a 423% *increase* in the number of measles cases[31]. The authorities blame the unvaccinated sections of the community for the rise in the incidence of measles, yet the studies available do not support these claims.

In 1985 the American government reported that 80% of notified cases of measles had been vaccinated[32]. In 1986 there was a measles epidemic at

Corpus Christi, Texas, in which 99% of the children affected had been vaccinated against measles, and over 95% were supposedly immune.[33]

A World Health Organisation study showed that in an unimmunised group of susceptible children the rate of contraction of measles was 2.4%, as compared to an immunised group in whom the rate was 33.5%.[34]

Do Vaccines Cause Harm to the Body?

Vaccinations can be directly responsible for conditions as mild as a sore throat, headache, fever or rash, to more severe conditions such as arthritis, paralysis, brain damage and death. The major problem with immunisation is the injection of foreign material directly into the bloodstream, without the normal assimilation and detoxification by the skin, mucous membranes or liver.

Anaphylactic shock

A vaccine preparation contains protein, bacterial and viral particles, sometimes live viruses as well as preservatives, neutralisers and carrying agents. Any person who collapses and dies, or who develops sudden, severe respiratory or skin symptoms within fifteen minutes to a day after taking a vaccine could be suffering from a personal sensitivity, i.e. an allergy to the poisonous contents of the vaccine.[35] This type of reaction is known as anaphylactic shock, and anyone administering vaccines is trained in the emergency procedures that are needed should this occur, as it is known that death can ensue very rapidly.

Neurological disorders

It is a fact that children have been brain damaged within a few days of being immunised. A recent study at the University of California estimates that as many as one in every thirteen children had persistent, high-pitched crying after the D.P.T. (diphtheria, pertussin and tetanus) vaccine, noting that .....'this may be indicative of brain damage'.[36]

Adverse reactions may be uncommon but such statistics are, more often than not, under reported. Doctors are reluctant to admit that there may be a causal relationship between neurological disorders and the administration of the vaccine. In the United States, a young boy died thirty-three hours after D.P.T. immunisation. The coroner denied any connection and wrote on his certificate 'death due to irreversible shock'. He said he was unable to implicate the vaccine .....'because the state's standing on immunisation would be in uproar'.[37]

Sudden infant death syndrome (SIDS)

The D.P.T. vaccine has been strongly linked with the advent of 'Sudden Infant Death Syndrome' (S.I.D.S.).[38] Dr. William Torch, of the Nevada School of Medicine, issued a report showing that two-thirds of 103 children who died of S.I.D.S. had been immunised with D.P.T. vaccine in the three weeks before their deaths, many dying within a day of the vaccine. He asserts that this was not mere coincidence and that a causal relationship is very likely.[39]

Cancer and auto-immune diseases

In the case of viral immunisation, the viral elements may persist in the blood for a long time after the injection, perhaps permanently. Viruses have the property of being able to attach their own genetic material to that of the 'host' cell. The host cell may then produce slightly abnormal proteins, which contain portions from the viral genetic material. This often causes an immune response of the cell against its own slightly abnormal proteins and hence the phenomena of auto-immune diseases (where the immune system attacks itself) such as cancer, leukaemia, rheumatoid arthritis, multiple sclerosis and lupus.

Acquired Immune Deficiency Syndrome (A.I.D.S.)

The smallpox vaccine has been linked to a number of phenomena concerning acquired immune deficiency syndrome (A.I.D.S.).[40]

The seven Central African states most affected by A.I.D.S. were the most intensively immunised states. Brazil, the only South American country covered in the immunisation campaign, had the highest incidence of A.I.D.S. About 14,000 Haitians who were with the United Nations armed services in Africa were covered in the immunisation programme. Haiti has one of the highest incidences of A.I.D.S., and is a popular resort among the homosexual men of San Francisco.

Dr. Richard Moskowitz states: 'Vaccines in fact only drive the disease deeper into the interior and cause us to harbour it chronically, with the result that our responses to disease become progressively weaker.'[41] This is typically the case with A.I.D.S. patients.

Defects in The Immunisation Theory

The theory of immunisation presupposes that the production of antibodies in response to the vaccine will protect the body when the 'real' disease comes along. However, it does not always seem to work that way.

For instance, agamma globulin-anaemic children are incapable of producing antibodies, yet they recover from measles and other infectious diseases almost as quickly as other children.

A study was carried out around the time of the diphtheria epidemic in 1950 and published by the British Medical Council,[42] which concluded that there was no relationship between antibody count and the incidence of disease. Researchers found resistant people with extremely low antibody counts and people who developed the disease with high counts. This study was abandoned because of the implications of the initial results.

Dr. Wendell Belfield, of San Jose, California, says that 'antibodies are not needed when the primary immunological defence is functioning at maximum capacity. Antibody production appears to occur *only if viruses survive the primary defence*'.[43]

Recent research suggests that the most effective systems for developing immunity are concerned with the skin, digestive and respiratory tracts, i.e. those systems involved with natural immunity, hence the recent interest in oral vaccines.

An injected vaccine tricks the body into no longer initiating a generalised inflammatory response, the virus being placed directly into the blood stream past the body's normal lines of defence and given access to the major organs and tissues. This elicits an antibody response, the very reaction that the body has evolved to produce *only as a last resort*. It is not an indication of a healthy immune response.

Research indicates that this immune reaction in response to vaccination substantially commits the immune cells to the specific antigens involved in the vaccine, so that they are incapable of reacting against other infections.[44] These findings indicate that our immunological reserve is substantially reduced, leading to a generally lowered resistance. The most serious charge against vaccinations and immunisations is the widespread and subtle long-term effects of an overloaded and damaged immune system.

Considering the above factors, it may be reasonable to suppose that an individual is reduced to a worse state of health after vaccination.

The Question of Cure

Within the system of orthodox medicine there are no criteria for 'cure' other than the removal of apparently related symptoms. Other forms of medicine have observed distinct patterns in the appearance of symptoms in diseased patients, comparing both treated and untreated individuals. Therapists now have definite criteria to use in assessing whether the treatment given is acting curatively or not.

For example, after orthodox treatment of eczema, it is very common for a patient to suffer from asthma. This is considered normal, or at least predictable, after 'curing' eczema. In other forms of medicine the disease can be said to have moved inwards, and the eczema has been suppressed. After, for example, homœopathic treatment of such asthma cases, the eczema often returns before the patient is healed, leaving no further symptoms.

Measles, mumps, and rubella among supposedly immune school children continue to be reported. These diseases, which are essentially benign self-limiting diseases of childhood, are being transformed by the use of vaccines into more severe diseases of adolescence and adulthood, with complications that include liver abnormalities, pneumonia and arthritis[45]. Could it be that the childhood illnesses are a very necessary process in the maturity of a person's immune system?

Chronic disease is now on the increase, cancer and auto-immune diseases are increasing at rates faster than the increase in life expectancy. The fact that people live longer now cannot account for the rise in chronic disease.[46]

A recent article in *The Guardian* claimed the first serious prospect of a 'cure' for A.I.D.S. in a patient treated with the drug A.Z.T. together with a bone marrow transplant.[47] Approximately 40 days after the transplant the patient died of a 'separate' lymphoma cancer, but *'The A.I.D.S. virus had been completely eradicated as shown by post mortem'* .....a cured case?

Why Do Doctors Continue to Immunise?

Much of orthodox medical practice rests on the germ theory of disease. Claiming success with antibacterial and antiviral treatments would justify this approach. However, the possibility that immunisation is ineffective and dangerous throws a substantial amount of orthodox treatment into doubt.

Many doctors are unwilling to face the inevitable consequences of such scrutiny, and, although some are, fewer still are willing to make public their findings. The dilemma faced by many can be illustrated by the following account.

Fourteen years after the measles vaccine was introduced, Los Angeles suffered a severe measles epidemic. Many physicians routinely gave measles vaccine to every child available, several did not. One Los Angeles physician who refused to vaccinate his own seven-month-old baby said 'I'm worried about what happens when the vaccine virus may not only offer little protection but may also stay around in the body, working in a way we don't know much about'.

Doctors know that viral elements, found in live vaccines, can emerge later in the form of encephalitis, multiple sclerosis, and as potential seeds for the development of cancer. The Los Angeles doctor rationalised his contradictory behaviour with the comment that....... 'as a parent I have the luxury of making a choice for my child. As a physician.....legally and professionally I have to accept the recommendations of the profession'.[48]

In the U.K. there is now the additional factor of financial incentives for doctors, to encourage them to achieve the highest possible immunisation 'targets'. This means that doctors who vaccinate the largest percentage of patients on their books stand to gain the most, whilst those who exercise greater discretion in the administration of vaccines, or who are willing to support parents who do not wish their children to be immunised are financially penalised.

Why Have Infectious Diseases Declined?

In the U.S.A. doctors admit that 40% of the population are not vaccinated against polio, yet where is polio? If immunisation can give us no immunity, where is our protection?

A recent World Health Organisation report shows that the disease and mortality rates in the Third World bear no correlation to the amount of money spent on medical treatment, including vaccination programmes, but are more closely related to the standard of hygiene and diet. It is suggested that these are the real reasons for the decline in infectious diseases world wide.[49]

Such declines have also been linked to a simple reclassification of diseases when occurring in vaccinated individuals, as is known to be the case with smallpox.

It is also likely that many infectious diseases which show a decline in incidence in the young tend to occur more frequently later on in life in a more potentially dangerous form.

Finally, as illustrated on page 28, studies have shown that infectious diseases have their own cycles of peak and decline which are largely unchanged by the introductions of immunisations and other medical treatments.

What are the Options?

Health is the only option - a healthy mind and body carries the best immunity. Creating an unnecessary fear of disease is futile and in itself can be as damaging as any life-threatening condition. The following are important considerations.

Environmental and Dietary Factors

The authorities in Leicester were led to try improved sanitation since their previous inoculation campaign of 1871 and 1872 appeared to have failed in the prevention of smallpox. Their largely unvaccinated population had the best health rate in all of the industrial towns of Great Britain. When compared to the smallpox deaths of the army and navy, at that time the most vaccinated sector of the public, the death rate in Leicester was almost half.[50]

Dr. Lincoln Graham, a naturopathic physician of the early part of this century, described how 28 cases of diphtheria were treated without a single fatality by fasting, drinking water and the use of enemas.[51]

According to the Journal of the American Medical Association 90 children with whooping cough were treated daily with vitamin C supplements. The children recovered within 20 days as compared to vaccine-treated individuals who took an average of 34 days to recover. When vitamin C was started in the catarrhal stages of the disease, in three-quarters of the cases, the spasmodic stage was wholly prevented.[52]

Iodine, calcium, potassium, and phosphorous supplements have been successfully used to prevent and treat various paralytic diseases including polio, herpes zoster, and encephalitis.

Therapies that Stimulate Health

The success of homœopathy and acupuncture in treating so-called incurable and infectious diseases is well documented.

In Naples in 1854-55, Dr. Rubini treated 225 cholera cases homœopathically without a single death. In London in 1854, the Homœopathic Hospital had a 16% death rate from cholera while the fatality rate in Chelsea under orthodox treatment was 54%. Dr. Dorothy Shepherd, practising in the 1950's and 60's, gave homœopathic medicines as preventatives for whooping cough to 364 children, some as young as two weeks old, and not one developed the disease.[53] Firsthand accounts can also be obtained from the many registered practitioners.

Establishing How Disease is Really Caused and Cured

Disease is an individual process relating to specific conditions and personal susceptibilities. It is not a hit-or-miss affair left to the discretion of attacking micro-organisms. Disorders resulting from infectious diseases become less likely as ones' level of health increases. The following analogy, although hypothetical, does serve to illustrate this point.

If a drug with its associated risks was to be developed for the prevention of lung cancer because statistics showed that one in 200 people die of this disease every year, then individuals might be persuaded to risk the harmful effects of the drug to avoid the disease.

However, if it later transpired that all deaths due to lung cancer occurred in individuals who had smoked cigarettes for a minimum of two years, then the risk of developing the disease would not apply to non-smokers. The most effective preventative measure would clearly be to avoid smoking, and any risks associated with the drug would present an unnecessary hazard to non-smokers. Everyone would then be in a position to make an informed decision, either to avoid smoking or to carry on and possibly take the drug.

This example is obviously an over-simplification as there will always be many factors that contribute to someone contracting a disease, including each individuals' particular weaknesses. However, it does illustrate the importance of understanding the many factors that give rise to disease.

A far greater proportion of the work of health authorities should include the careful analysis of such factors. This empowers individuals with the knowledge and the option to stay healthy or to risk illness. Serious disorders are *not* statistical probabilities for all to fear equally, but are the result of a certain combination of factors that may, often with hindsight, prove to be avoidable.

With regard to any therapy, it is not enough to remove symptoms of one disease only to replace them with those of another. Therefore, in assessing the effects of any medical treatment, the total health of the patient needs to be analysed for as long a time period as possible. Symptoms that do not appear to be related to the original complaint may later show strong correlations to the *treatment* given. Careful evaluation of such results will reveal the true nature of the treatment as being either curative or degenerative.

Summary and Conclusions

The assumptions of the original researchers into disease can be summarised as follows: micro-organisms are directly responsible for disease, and in destroying them and avoiding contamination we may combat disease and hence improve health. These assumptions have been proved wrong.

Micro-organisms are a result of ill-health, therefore increasing ones level of health should be of the foremost concern. This can be achieved by improving the nutritional quality of our diet, reducing our intake of toxins from the environment, optimising physical function and psychological stability through appropriate exercise and employing stimulatory therapies such as acupuncture, homoeopathy, osteopathy, herbalism and naturopathy.

The assumptions of the original researchers into vaccines can be summarised as follows: the presence of antibodies to micro-organisms indicates a level of immunity to the associated infectious disease, therefore stimulating antibody production increases health and immunity. These assumptions have been proved wrong.

The antibody response is the last in a long line of defence mechanisms, and initiating this response artificially through immunisation depletes the body's immune reserve and increases susceptibility to disease.

Immunity can be very effectively obtained without the production of blood antibodies.

Antimicrobial techniques may be necessary when all else fails, but most alternative therapists operate exclusively without them, preferring to promote and maintain health rather than destroying the supposed agents of disease.

Immunisation has developed from a theory of disease and immunity that has serious flaws. The evidence suggests that they are responsible for widespread degeneration in peoples health, and that natural immunity is far safer and more effective.

The Questions Remain

Since the introduction of immunisations many publications have warned of their dangers and possible ineffectiveness, giving detailed results of research and interviews with patients and parents of vaccine damaged children. Harris Coulter states that there has been no official reaction to the very serious charges made in his book *D.P.T. - A Shot in the Dark?* Why do the authorities choose to ignore the criticisms?

The Health Department in the U.K. publish evidence for the efficacy of immunisations, including graphs showing the decline in incidence and death rates of certain diseases from the 1950's onwards, stating that these reductions have been due to the introduction of immunisations.[54] Why do they not publish figures showing the rates of decline that were occurring *before* the 1950's, when no vaccines were available?[55]

England & Wales: Deaths of children under 15 years attributed to scarlet fever, diphtheria, whooping cough and measles (Porter, 1971).

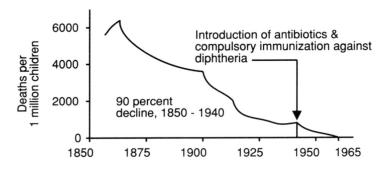

Population statistics without controls contain so many variables that worthwhile conclusions are very difficult to make. Why have vaccine producers failed to conduct long-term scientific trials testing the safety and effectiveness of immunisations as compared to naturally acquired immunity?

It can take many years to die of a serious disease, it can take equally as long for the effects of medical procedures to manifest as recognisable disease symptoms. Why should there be a limit from the time of immunisation after which symptoms cannot be attributable to the vaccine? Typical examples are just 72 hours for the whooping cough vaccine and 8-20 days for the live vaccines of measles, mumps, rubella and polio.[56]

If, after immunisation against measles, for example, individuals are more likely to contract serious disorders such as meningitis, cancer and multiple sclerosis, and are less likely to contract measles, should a decrease in measles notifications be used in measuring the effectiveness of the vaccine?

Does the immunisation issue have implications beyond that of simply testing the efficacy of a medical procedure? Perhaps the time has come for these unanswered questions to be raised and publically debated.

Recommended Reading

Walene James
Immunisation: The reality behind the myth
Bergin and Garvey Inc., USA, 1988

Leon Chaitow
Vaccinations and Immunisations - Dangers, Delusions and Alternatives
C.W. Daniel, Saffron Walden, Essex, 1987

E.D. Hume
Pasteur Exposed
Bookreal, W.A., Australia, 1989

R. Neustaedter
The Immunisation Decision: A guide for parents
North Atlantic books, California, 1990

H.L. Coulter and B.L. Fisher
D.P.T. - A Shot In The Dark
Avery Publishing Group, New York, 1987

H.L. Coulter
Vaccination, Social Violence and Criminality
North Atlantic Books, California 1990

R. Moskowitz
The Case Against Immunisations
The Society of Homoeopaths, 2 Artizan Rd., Northampton NN1 4HU

U. K. Department of Health
Immunisation Against Infectious Disease
HMSO Publications, 1990

References

1   E.D. Hume
    Pasteur Exposed - The False Foundations of Modern Medicine
    Bookreal, Australia, 1989

2   *Journal of the Franklin Institute*
    U.S.A., February 1944, p. 117

3   W. James
    Immunisation, The Reality behind the Myth

4   *Scientific American*
    April, 1955, p. 98

5   W. James
    op. cit.

6   Statistics presented at the *Presidential Address of the British Association
    for the Advancement of Sciences*
    Porter, 1971

7   *Organic Consumer Report*
    California, March 11th, 1975

8   E.D. Hume
    op. cit.

9   *The Guardian*
    London, 25th November 1991

10 W. James
    op. cit.

11 Organic Consumer Report
    California, March 11th, 1975

12 R. Mendelson M.D.
    How to raise a healthy child in spite of your doctor
    Contemporary Books Inc., Chicago, Illinois, 1984

13 E.D. Hume
    op. cit., p. 172

14 E. D. Hume
    op. cit., p. 174

15 E. D. Hume
    op. cit.

16 W. James
    op. cit, p. 32

17 W. James
    op. cit.

18 H.L. Coulter and B.L. Fisher
    DPT - A Shot in the Dark
    Warner Books Inc., New York

19 W. James
    op. cit.

20 *The Health Crisis*
    The Natural Medicines Society

21 William Howard Hay M.D.
    The House of Representatives Congressional Record
    December 21st, 1937, U.S.A.

22 P. Airola N.D., PhD.
    Everywomans Book
    Health Plus, Phoenix, Arizona

23 R. Mendelson M.D.
    The People's Doctor Immunisation Report (ii), Vol. 4

24 P. Airola
    op. cit., p. 227

25 R. Mendelson
    How to Raise a healthy Child

26 R. Mendelson
    op. cit.

27 What Doctors Don't Tell You
    The WDDTY Vaccination Handbook
    The Wallace Press 1991

28   WDDTY
     Op. cit.
29   WDDTY
     Op. cit., p. 25
30   *Development of Biological Standards*, Vol. 432
     S. Kruger, Basel, 1979
31   WDDTY
     Op. cit., p. 2
32   Centre for Disease Control Morbidity and Mortality Weekly Report
     6th June 1986, U.S.A.
33   New England Journal of Medicine
     26th March 1987, U.S.A.
34   P. Airola
     op. cit., p. 279
35   W. James
     op. cit.
36   W. James
     op. cit.
37   H.L. Coulter and B. L. Fisher
     op. cit.
38   H.L. Coulter and B. L. Fisher
     op. cit.
39   R. Mendelson M.D.
     op. cit.
40   W. James
     op. cit., p. 102
41   R. Moskowitz M.D.
     The Case Against Immunisations
     Journal of the American Institute of Homœopathy, Vol. 76, March 1983
42   British Medical Council
     Publication 272, May 1950
43   G. Dettman PhD. and A. Kalokerinos M.D.
     The Dangers of Immunisation
     Biological Research Institute, Victoria, Australia, 1979
44   Arthur Research Corporation
     Arizona
45   W. James
     Op. cit., p. 34
46   Natural Medicines Society
     op. cit.
47   *The Guardian*
     London, 20th December 1989
48   R. Mendelson M.D.
     op. cit.
49   Natural Medicines Society
     op. cit.
50   E. D. Hume
     op. cit., p. 173
51   W. James
     op. cit.
52   *Journal of the American Medical Association*
     November 4th 1950
53   Dr. Dorothy Shepherd
     Homœopathy in Epidemic Diseases
     C. W. Daniel Co. Ltd., Saffron Walden, Essex
54   *Immunisation Against Infectious Disease*
     H.M.S.O., 1990
55   W. James
     op. cit., p. 25
56   The Association for Parents of Vaccine-Damaged Children
     2 Church Street, Warwickshire, CV36 4AP